WEIGHT LOSS SOLUTION

Practical steps to loosing weight; all about dieting and weight loss

By

Joshua Oguledo

Copyright @2022 Joshua Oguledo

TABLE OF CONTENT

INTRODUCTION

The recipe for shedding pounds is basic: eat less and practice more.

In any case, it's not exactly all that basic, right?

Long haul weight reduction isn't incomprehensible, however you in all actuality do need to be committed.

Having a weight reduction plan for your prosperity is a decent beginning. The following are ten things that ought to go into your weight reduction plan.

1. Have breakfast. This holds you back from getting excessively ravenous later and afterward,

letting completely go over what you decide to eat later in the day.

2. Stock your fridge and storage space with good food varieties and tidbits and cutoff

high-fat, high-salt snacks, for example, potato chips and treats.

3. Top off on Fiber. Eat food sources like natural products, vegetables and entire grains. The strands in these food sources will top you off leaving less space for undesirable decisions.

4. Try not to fall into negative behavior patterns on ends of the week. Many individuals will follow a severe diet on ends of the week just to fall once more into eating more (undesirable) on the ends

of the week as a compensation for "being great" throughout the week. Sadly, this can

make you recover the weight you might have lost during the week.

5. Watch segment sizes. Your impression of what a serving size ought to be and a "valid" serving size can contrast emphatically. Measure your parts precisely, particularly when you initially start your good dieting system.

6. Put forth way of life objectives - not weight reduction objectives. Obligation to practicing good eating habits

food sources prompts sound weight reduction - bit by bit. Checking your weight out day to day can cause debilitation and will make many individuals surrender and go back to undesirable food decisions.

7. Take solid snacks with you when you go on street outings. Get sound granola bars, bananas, apples and other natural product to forestall the enticement of halting for a treat or milk shake.

8. Try not to deny yourself the food sources you love. In the event that you totally love chocolate, feel free to have a little piece - a big part of a sweet treat rather than an entirety.

Consuming less calories and Weight reduction one! Also, try not to eat your "goes a little overboard" consistently. Save them for when you truly need them!

9. Begin moving. Practice is the way to long haul weight reduction. You've heard

the expression, "Get out of the way." Excessively evident!

10. Keep a diary. Recording what you eat, when and the amount you practice and your mind-sets will keep you on target and spurred to proceed the course.

Weight reduction is accomplished by both eating routine and exercise. It is likewise accomplished by diligence. If you "tumble off the cart" at some point, get yourself and proceed with your sound way of life the following.

Try not to surrender!

CHAPTER 1:

A COUPLE OF STRAIGHTFORWARD TIPS TO LOSE WEIGHT

Weight reduction is an extreme outcome to get paying little heed to weight or even out

of actual wellness. There are various ways of getting more fit, some more unfortunate than others, however the ones that work are most times the most convoluted to pull off.

Certain individuals might prescribe eating less to get more fit, and at times eating less is a critical part of shedding pounds, however generally speaking, eating is

a need if one wishes to bring down their own weight.

Without food and the calories, they supply, your body has no energy to consume

furthermore, thus will transform your current muscle into fat. To get in shape,

you should sincerely commit a responsibility, a responsibility that should not be broken if

you want results.

Try not to misjudge this for the possibility that you can never enjoy during your diet, yet be certain that you have drawn sensible lines for yourself that you are prepared to focus on. In the event that you are on a severe eating regimen, a "cheat" feast here

furthermore, there will go quite far to keeping you blissful.

To find lasting success in accomplishing your objective of weight reduction: set various, more modest, all the more effectively achievable objectives for yourself. These will keep you self-inspired

furthermore, bound to getting your general objective of a more joyful and better life.

10 Weight reduction Tips

1. Consume a bigger number of calories than you consume. Assuming this makes you go: "D-uuuh!!", wake up and think about that this rudimentary part of eating fewer carbs get away incalculable confused - and destined - health food nuts. Tabloids might profess to have the "marvel food varieties" that will permit you to eat like a pig and have the pounds soften off, however it's a heap.

2. Lay out your base digestion, and put forth an objective calorie objective approx. 500

calories beneath it. I composed an article committed to laying out your.

Slimming down and Weight reduction

digestion prior, so find it in the article chronicle in the event that you really want a

boost.

3. Keep a genuine log. Make appraisals of the number of calories you that stuff

yourself with each dinner and count up the absolute to ensure you stay inside

your objective calorie objective. Advantageous "botches," under-gauges and absent mindedness permits you to eat all the more

currently, however you're overcoming the entirety

reason behind consuming less calories.

4. Effectively pick great wellsprings of fat. This

might seem like dumb guidance - -

shouldn't you Stay away from fat while

consuming less calories? Indeed, yes and negative.

You need to keep

consuming some fat, simply not getting carried

away. Stay away from margarine, bacon, entirety

milk, coconuts and such like the plague. All

things being equal, utilize olive oil (virgin) and

greasy fish.

Peanut butter is an intriguing subject. I used to place it in a similar class as the "awful" fats. It has a place there, pressing immersed fat as well as course stopping up trans unsaturated fats. Be that as it may, in view of profoundly informal declarations by others as well as private experience, it appears to be a small bunch of peanuts every so often while eating less junk food can do ponders in keeping energy steps up while not unleashing ruin with your general eating regimen. Odd and unreasonable? You betcha. Yet, it just so ends up working in any case, similar to honey bees flying however they in fact ought not be ready to.

5. Eat little however regular dinners over the course of the day. You've heard it 1,000,000 times, I'm certain, yet realities stay: to keep an even degree of blood sugar, you need to eat little, adjusted feasts.

6. Try not to go weak on the power lifting. At the point when you diet, you're in the peril zone for losing bulk more often than not. To stay away from this, keeping

siphoning iron, and be determined about it!

7. Keep away from liquor. Considering that grill season has arrived, this can be extreme

at the point when your companions draw out the super cold brew-skis. The arrangement is straightforward:

Just partner with different jocks, so you essentially will not be the solitary

dweeb tasting an eating routine pop! For those of you who have the absurd thought

that your life shouldn't spin around lifting weights: Wake up.

8. Hit the treadmill with some restraint. Completing 45 minutes on the stair master consistently is an incredible method for getting the pounds off speedier.

Eating less junk food and Weight reduction

bound to begin losing bulk. When and how much

is individual (and contingent upon what you've

needed to eat before in the day) however stay

away from cardio

meetings more than 60 minutes. Assuming that

you want the discipline do one meeting in the

morning and one at night. Likewise make sure to

remain in the 65%-70%

pulse zone for ideal fat consume.

9. Plan "cheating" days to remain normal.

Abstaining from excessive food intake is

unpleasant. Regardless of how gung-ho and

persuaded you are the point at which you begin,

you'll have days when everything is murkiness

and the world is on a mission to get you. Try to get a treat once seven days on a set day (Saturday is great) as it gives you something to anticipate.

A succulent burger is greasy and calorie-thick, however on the off chance that you plan by doing extra

cardio for three days ahead of time you'll come in accurate for the week.

10. Try not to fear soy. I used to keep away from counterfeit meat items, however having been hitched to a veggie lover for 3+ years I've attempted soy wieners, burgers,

chicken patties, even rib-lets that taste very much like the genuine article. Also, here's the kicker: Soy items is for the most part protein!

Truly, soy protein isn't the greatest out there, however in the event that you drink a

glass of milk or have some other excellent protein source with it you can

knock up the general quality in a rush. Furthermore, soy has various extraordinary

medical advantages when eaten with some restraint and contains almost no fat.

CHAPTER 2

FAT CONSUMING FOOD VARIETIES

What number of time did You search for the marvel nourishment for weight reduction? Perhaps with fascinating name and extravagant look?

Indeed, perhaps you're failing to remember those usually accessible food varieties, frequently underestimated yet top notch concerning detox and digestion sponsor characteristics. here is a rundown of 19 of them!

1.Garlic. Heaps of minerals, catalysts and amino

acids; Nutrients A, B1, B2,

B6, B12, C, D. Just 41 KCAL per 100 grams.

Reactivates Your digestion while keeping the

cholesterol to shake low levels.

2. Banana. Sugars with little fats. Calcium, Iron,

Magnesium, Potassium,

Nutrients: A, C, Tannin and Serotonin. Just 66

Kcal per 100 grams. An extraordinary

hunger suppressant nibble.

3. Onion. Rich of Nutrients A, C, E, and of B

gathering of nutrients. Too,

Potassium, Calcium, Sodium; help diuretic action

and an incredible cellulite

warrior. Assists with keeping blood sugars corrals.

4. Drug grass. Not much utilized in the present nourishment, but rather an extraordinary companion of

weight reduction. Helps controlling fats consumption.

5. Strawberry. Low Sugars, Minerals and L-ascorbic acid rich. Just 27 KCAL per

100 grams.

6. Corn Chips. However, grains, Vegetables blended. Helps a ton Your

digestion and just 14 KCAL per 100 grams.

7. Kiwi. Potassium rich and Calcium, Iron, Zinc as well.

8. Salad. Rich of strands and extremely poor in calories (just 14 KCAL per 100 grams); diuretic capabilities and craving suppressant, because of huge volume/low KCAL proportion. Parcel of minerals as well.

9. Lemon. Least sugar content for a similar natural product family (just 2,3%), rich

in Nutrients and just 11 KCAL per 100 grams. Helps blood course and battles cellulitis.

10. Apple. L-ascorbic acid, Potassium, Magnesium, fantastic elevated cholesterol contender.

11. Nut. Plentiful in Fats, Proteins, Sugars and Nutrients. Helps Fat Consuming on account of good Calcium + Magnesium contents.

12. Wheat. Just 319 KCAL per 100 grams and extremely wealthy in Proteins, Amino

acids, Iron, Calcium, Potassium and Magnesium. Yet additionally, great substance of Nutrients. Helps diuretic works and battles close to home eating.

13. Chicken. White meat, low fat substance, limits admission of fats, sodium and

cholesterol.

14. Rocla Salad. Incredible substance of Vitamin A and C, and extraordinary Digestion promoter. Just 16 KCAL per 100 grams.

15. Soy. Wealthy in Proteins and Folic Corrosive. Battles Weight acquiring and makes a difference re-balancing digestion.

16. Tea. contains fat consuming caffeine, minerals and B Gathering Nutrients. Invigorate Digestion and has a 0 Calories consumption.

17. Egg. Hyperphrenic food. Loads of Minerals and Proteins, helps groom nonfat mass which is critical to increment muscle to fat ratio' consuming.

18. Wine. Contains cell reinforcement substances that assist with safeguarding the heart and battle maturing.

19. Pumpkin. Plentiful in vitamin B, C, E Nutrients, minerals and just 18 KCAL per 100 grams. Helped diuretic capabilities.

CHAPTER 3

AM I LANGUID?

Is the explanation that there has been an expansion in stoutness due to the reality that grown-ups in the present society are lethargic?

Are we as a whole a lot of lazy habitual slouches that sit idle be that as it may, lounge around and eat constantly? I say no. Rather we are a result of our progressive, mechanical society.

I'm not saying we can fault innovation, rather I'm expressing that as with our childhood, the grown-ups are likewise an impression of the general public that encompasses them. It's anything but a reason, however it is an idea I considered in view of my commonplace day.

I get up in the first part of the day, not to an exasperating buzz, signal, or the blasting of the radio. These cautions would get my blood hustling right from the beginning, yet I would hit rest to stop the madness. Then it would work out once more, and once more, the rest bar. After a couple of seasons of this I would now be behind schedule for work, hurry to the

shower on the off chance that I even had time, hurry to the vehicle, and dash off to work. Not in the present world. All things considered, I wake to the relieving sound of the sea on my Homeric's radio and gradually wake calmly. No blood siphoning, no expanded pulse. I simply have a quite sluggish, simple arousing. Then, I head to the shower where I put go on my shower Album player and pay attention to something that I appreciate while I take as much time as necessary letting the water

nearly run cold. During my drying off and getting dressed time of the morning, I can

hear my espresso being made on the espresso producer that is set to make me a cup each day with me not doing a thing. While I

sit and drink my espresso contemplating the day

in front of me, I notice that it is practically gone,

so I tenderly press a button on my key ring that

begins my vehicle and gets it decent and

warm for me before I even get to it.

I can then go for my relaxed walk to my vehicle,

get in, and have a decent serene

drive to work (except any unexpected

uncontrollable anger). In no way like before when

I needed to hurry to my vehicle since I was late

more often than not due to the disturbance of my

caution or run since it was cold and afterward get

in and shake

what's more, shudder for 10 minutes until it

heated up. When at work I end up taking out my

PDA and it is on me to see what

plan for the afternoon. No, no seriously flipping

through pages of my pocket schedule or scheduler.

My work day is straightforward and unremarkable,

yet rather than running ever changing through the

workplace to receive messages to

everybody, I can now just send an official email

with the push of a

button. At the point when the time has come to

leave, I again start my vehicle from my office and

commute home.

Showing up at home, I put in a microwave supper

that doesn't need to be

slashed up, cut up, mixed, mixed, worked, jabbed,

or even pushed. Press a couple of buttons and

after five minutes I'm sitting before the television

watching the shows I recorded on my link's

computerized recorder and eating my five-minute,

nuked dinner. Could I have done this previously?

The response is no, on the grounds that I would

have

needed to genuinely make something to eat, and

there wouldn't be anything on Television worth

watching, so I would eat and go follow through

with something like yard work, clean the house,

play with the children, whatever, simply another thing to possess the time. Oh no, while I was eating, I got a few pieces on the floor and afterward dropped an erring on the way back to the kitchen. Anyway, I will simply press the button on my robot vacuum cleaner and let it clean the entire floor as it is prearranged to do. At long last, my day is reaching a conclusion and on second thought of accomplishing something, truth be told helpful before I hit the hay, I can't avoid the chance to surf the Web for a brief period, perhaps talk to certain companions or family members, and check my email. Plus, I need to connect my PDA to the PC in any case. Presently my languid or mechanically useless day is finished.

This entire story takes me back to my inquiry that began the entire thing.

Am I lethargic or am I simply a result of my current circumstance. It is this creator's assessment that I am both. A long time back, even the basic things like making the supper would be work out, yet presently it is too simple since it is finished for you in a container.

All that today is simple and most grown-ups are on the weighty side, on the grounds that things are more straightforward and don't take as much energy. That doesn't mean we in the society are apathetic, it implies we don't need to endeavor as

a lot to achieve the ordinary necessary schedules

to finish the day.

Notwithstanding, I could come by the center

returning, or take a stroll later

supper, so I'm likewise sluggish as well. The Web

simply pulls me in many evenings

also, I just can't cause myself to do anything more

after supper. Disgrace on

your innovation for holding that firearm to my

head.

CHAPTER 4

DO ALL DIETS WORK?

Have you shed pounds in the past just to recapture it a brief time frame later?

Have you followed each diet including Atkins, South Ocean side, the Drinking Man's eating regimen, the Peanut Butter diet, or even the Chocolate Diet?

These weight control plans work, and not a solitary one of them work, meaning you can and most likely get in shape on any of them, however you won't keep it off. What difference would it make?

Since the day will come when the eating regimen is finished and you're right back to

your standard daily practice; the very normal that got you fat in any case.

In the past weight control plans conveyed an admonition not to remain on them longer than the endorsed period; generally two weeks, exactly a simple three days. The present well known counts calories are endeavoring to style themselves as way of life decisions, yet all the same this isn't working all things considered.

Individuals need to have the option to eat a sandwich from time to time. They need the burger and the bun! Make progress toward balance picking food varieties you like, and you'll have a superior opportunity to last weight reduction achievement.

Little Changes: Huge Response to Weight reduction Blues Begin today, and work each day in turn making a couple of little changes

for example, changing to the sans calorie soda pops then, at that point, weaning yourself down to two or less a day (in the event that you drink more than that now obviously).

Changes don't need to be exceptional. Attempting to roll out extreme improvements in, as a matter of fact

your way of life never works on the grounds that while you might be blissful at the outset, you gradually become hopeless around the end. That is the issue right, truth be told there: you expect an end.

Weight reduction Comes Down to Decisions Converse with individuals who've shed pounds and kept it off. They'll say, "This is a way of life." It's about decisions you make consistently. Are you deciding to take an additional aiding, despite the fact that you're easily full? Change that one conduct and you're coming. Do you decide to take the sack of chips to the love seat? Change that, truth be told quit eating on the sofa completely and you're one bit nearer. Take out the propensity for snatching a couple of chomps on your far beyond the sweets dish, that by itself can shave a few pounds. I once lost eight pounds basically by disposing of the treats dish I kept at my work area (not to notice the cash I saved not several pounds of treats seven days).

Pick each little propensity or conduct in turn, not your whole presence, and you'll have a vastly improved opportunity to arrive at your weight

reduction objectives.

CHAPTER 5

A STRAIGHTFORWARD ARRANGEMENT FOR WEIGHT REDUCTION

The math is straightforward. One pound of fat equivalents 3500 calories.

Need to lose a pound seven days?

Then, at that point, you really want to consume 3500 calories less each week than you use. That is around 500 calories per day. By removing 500 calories per day from your typical everyday eating routine, while keeping your movement level something similar, you can lose roughly one pound seven days.

OK - that doesn't seem like a lot, particularly on the off chance that you're more than 25 pounds overweight. Many examinations has shown, however, that those individuals who get thinner progressively - at a pace of 1-2 pounds each week - are undeniably more prone to keep the load off and keep an ordinary load for a lifetime.

So how much precisely ARE 500 calories? Assuming you will lessen your everyday consumption by 500 calories, it assists with understanding what you want to remove, isn't that so?

This is the how simple it is to lose 500 calories per day:

• Use milk rather than cream in your espresso. Investment funds? 50 calories for every cup.

• Skirt the spread on your heated potato. Reserve funds? 100 calories

• Drink natural product seasoned water rather than a 16-ounce pop. Reserve funds? 200 calories

• Skirt the Huge Macintosh and have a plate of mixed greens all things considered. A Major Macintosh tips the scales at a walloping 460 calories. A new plate of mixed greens with a light dressing? Not exactly 100! Reserve funds? 360 calories.

• Pass by the sack of potato chips. A typical bite size pack of chips has north of 300 calories. Reserve funds? 300 calories

• Eat your corn on the ear. A 1 cup serving of canned corn has 165 calories. An ear of corn has 85. Investment funds? 80 calories.

• Change to low-fat cream cheddar on your bagel. Reserve funds? 90 calories per ounce.

• Love those chips and can't surrender them? Trade the thin fries out for thick steak-cut ones. Dainty French fries retain more oil than the thicker, meatier ones. Reserve funds? 50 calories for each 4 ounces serving.

Assuming you'd prefer take a gander at shedding pounds according to an activity viewpoint, you can likewise lose one pound seven days by increasing your action level by 500 calories a day. How simple is that to do? Investigate:

Go for a half-hour stroll around the recreation area. Go for the gold that is somewhat quicker than a walk, yet not quickly enough to be short of breath. Consume: 160 calories.

• Get out your bicycle and take a ride. Tackle a couple of moderate slopes and point for around five miles absolute. Consume: 250 calories

• Go out - and truly DANCE. The more you're out on the floor rather than at the table drinking as high as possible calorie drinks, the more you'll receive in return. Moving that makes you winded and heats up your body will get you a decent calorie investment funds. Consume: 400 calories for one hour

• Swimming is perfect for you, and loads of tomfoolery, as well. The water opposition implies you consume more calories, and you stay away from the pressure influence on joints from heart stimulating exercise, moving or strolling. Do a couple of laps at a sluggish creep - in the event that you can get as long as an hour you'll do perfect! Consume: 510 calories

• Get out into your nursery. An hour of planting undertakings that incorporates bowing and extending can wreck to however many calories as a lively walk. Consume: 250 calories.

• Play a round of tennis. Connect with a companion for a week after week tennis match-up also, you'll be flabbergasted at the distinction. One hour of enthusiastic tennis is one of the most incredible calorie burners around. Consume: 800 calories.

It's essential to remember that all activity/calorie numbers depend on

a lady weighing 130 pounds. Assuming you weigh more, you'll consume more. Need a special reward to consuming activity? At the

point when you work out, you construct muscle

by changing over it from fat. Three suppositions

which sort of body tissue consumes more calories

- in any event, when you're not working out. You

got it -

your body utilizes more energy to keep up with

and feed muscle than it fats.

For best outcomes, blend and coordinate food

reserve funds in with practices that consume

calories. Do remember that eating under 1000

calories every day for more

than a couple of days will persuade your body that

it's destitute and slow your

digestion.

Keep calorie ranges sensible, and counsel a specialist on the off chance that you need a faster, more intense weight reduction.

CHAPTER 6

TAKING ON A LOW CARB DIET

Eats less carbs have showed up in a wide range of structures, particularly craze consumes less calories.

Among the issues with these prevailing fashion abstains from food that as well as frequently leaving you feeling exceptionally hungry they can likewise be undesirable and as it were work for a short space of time.

Research has shown that the best eating regimens are those that can be stuck to over extensive stretches of time. On account of trend eats less carbs, weight tends to be exceptionally sporadic and keeping in mind that you might get in shape at first it is actually normal to set that load back on and in the long run increment on your weight. One of the immense advantages of a low carb diet is that you don't have to feel hungry. This might seem like it maintains a strategic distance from the place of an eating regimen, however it doesn't. The point of consuming less calories isn't to eat less yet to shed pounds or eat all the more strongly. The generally renowned of all low carb abstains from food is the Atkins diet and this stays well known since it permits you to eat great measured feasts and is demonstrated to assist you with losing weight.

The rudiments of a low carb diet are that you can eat as much food as you like

until you are full, the length of you just eat the permitted food sources. For the most part talking, this incorporates meat, cheddar, fish, eggs and poultry. You are too

permitted a specific measure of green vegetables every day. As well similar to a solid method for getting thinner, a low carb diet will give you a supported weight misfortune meaning you can keep on getting more fit even after the underlying push and you will keep the load off whenever it is no more.

It will likewise bring down your cholesterol and circulatory strain along with balance out your glucose level. You ought to enhance a low carb diet with multi nutrients since your body will turn out to be somewhat kept from these fundamental nutrients.

Now that we've covered those parts of starches, how about we go to some of different elements that should be thought of. It has been assessed that three out of each and every four overweight individuals are dependent on starches. In any case, what's the significance here? Generally, it implies that you have a lot of the chemical insulin in your framework. This insulin prompts you to eat frequently and to eat some unacceptable kinds of food sources. Some of the indications of starch compulsion incorporate weariness, temperament swings, what's more, headaches which can be brought about by low glucose. A carb habit can lead you to consume an entire sack of pretzels at one sitting, or to enjoy a portion of a cake at supper time. Your body is adapted to eat however many carbs as could be expected under the circumstances. In this manner, it might appear to be that on occasion you're never truly fulfilled — regardless of how much or how frequently you eat.

On the authority Carb Junkies plan, you eat two dinners made out of vegetables what's more, protein; the other feast comprises of protein, vegetables that are not filled with starch, and carbs. During this last dinner, known as the award feast, you might actually eat dessert. Try to avoid the carbs for two dinners every day.

The creators of the program trust that, assuming you follow this routine, you will

lose your desires for carbs in time. If your desire to consume carbs doesn't vanish constantly seven day stretch of the program, they suggest really taking a look at your eating routine to see whether you are following the program intently.

With the Carb Fiends plan, as other eating regimen plans, you want to screen intently your part measures. Your diligent effort will be all to no end in the event that you permit yourself to revel in desserts — regardless of whether it is for only one dinner daily. Additionally, you need to ensure that the protein you consume isn't high in fat. You may need to eat fish, chicken with the skin eliminated, or lean meats while attempting to get a protein source.

One more significant part of the Carb Fiends plan is that you are not allowed fake sugar besides during your award dinner. This can be all in all a test, particularly in the event that you're familiar with improved espresso in the morning. Notwithstanding, it tends to be definitely worth the hardship over the long haul as you see those pounds soften away. There is no set time for the prize dinner; in any case, the creators of the arrangement suggest that the feast happen at night. This is on the grounds that it would be able require 12 to 24 hours for the body to conquer carb over-burden. There

is likewise a mental benefit to having the feast around evening time. It gives you

something to anticipate the entire day.

You ought to start your prize feast with a serving of mixed greens, like a Caesar salad or an Oriental serving of mixed greens, then partition the remainder of the dinner into thirds: 33% ought to comprise of low - carb vegetables, 33% protein, and 33% carbs. This recipe has demonstrated fruitful in empowering people to accomplish long haul weight reduction.

Similarly as with numerous other feast designs, the greatest test for the people who are on the Carb Fiends Diet is the capacity to stay with it. Eating less junk food can be difficult work, regardless of what sort of remunerations anticipate a person by the day's end.

Your responsibility will empower you to remain with the program, in any event, when it turns out to be especially difficult.

Surf the Internet, and you'll find various tributes offering gleaming audits of the Carb Fiends Diet. However, you ought to remember that

results can vary from one person to another. While certain individuals could see

fast weight reduction with the Carb Junkies plan, others might see just moderate

weight reduction. The outcome of the program might rely upon your own person

physiology.

Is the Carb Fiends Diet a craze? Everything relies upon who you converse with. While some individuals see it as a critical dietary leap forward, others view it as a fleeting curiosity. Clinical specialists differ concerning whether the Carb Fiends Diet

addresses sound nourishment. Eventually, you, in conference with your individual doctor, should conclude whether the Carb Junkies Diet will work for you.

The day will come when you can utilize something you read about here to have a useful effect. Then, at that point, you'll be happy you found opportunity to find out more about sugars.

CHAPTER 7

DETOX DIETS

Detox Diets are the last frenzy in eating less junk food, that is the reason the quantity of individuals looking for detox abstains from food is developing consistently.

You might have caught wind of poisons, detoxification, purging, cleaning; they

are completely connected with detox slims down.

Poisons are hurtful synthetics influencing your body. They are surrounding you (in your food, water, air) and inside you (as byproducts of digestion).

Your body kills most poisons and the rest are put away inside muscle versus fat.

These put away poisons joined with pressure can influence your well being in very disagreeable ways:

• Weight gain.

• Cerebral pains.

• Sensations of weariness and shortcoming.

• Acid reflux.

• Sore muscles and skin.

• Joint agonies.

These side effects will blur when you start detox.

All things considered, you might feel some distress in the absolute first days, however that is a typical body response.

You might feel cerebral pain or sore muscles, however that is on the grounds that the poisons are delivered quicker than your body can dispense with them. These side effects will not happen once more on the off-chance that you detox consistently.

Detoxification is the most common way of delivering and ousting the put away poisons through the disposal organs of your body - the digestion tracts, liver, lungs, kidneys and skin.

Detox and Disease Prevention

Detox Diets are dietary nutritious plans that utilization detoxification, which makes a difference you get more fit by purifying out your body and working on your digestion.

Detox Diets are prescribed for further developing protection from sickness, mental state, processing, fortifies the organs associated with detox.

Detox food

Detox Diets can assist with forestalling serious infections like disease, ADD, ADHD,

persistent weariness condition and different compound responsive qualities, as well as treat coronary illness, fibromyalgia, immune system sickness.

Detox Food varieties

Detox Diets suggest utilization of food varieties that are useful for your

well-being and vital for weight reduction - natural food sources, products of the soil.

You ought to hydrate and scale back handled food varieties, as well as surrender liquor and smoking. It would be ideal for you to be aware.

Detox Diets are very prohibitive and when you start a detox diet, you ought to follow it rigorously. Detox Diets are protected, however you ought to counsel your primary care physician prior to beginning.

Kinds of Detox Diets:

• **Fasting** - drinking just water, juices or stocks, or eating one sort of nourishment for a specific time frame. Your body begins consuming fat for energy.

- **Healthful enhancements** - admission of nutritious powders, nutrients and bundled protein snacks.

- **Hydrotherapy** - detoxifying through your skin pores by taking extraordinary showers.

- **Explicit detox counts calories** - last somewhere in the range of 7 and 30 days; there are fast detox abstains from food for oneself and three days, and long detox eats less carbs for a considerable length of time.